Staying with Me

Diane McShane

ISBN-13: 978-1502549600
ISBN-10: 1502549603

This book is dedicated to Joy.
Yes, that's my Mum, "Joy".
She taught me I do not have to accept pain.
I do not have to accept an outdated belief system
based on guilt, suffering and punishment.
That I can choose a path of peaceful surrender.
That life is for living in Joy
and when that Joy can no longer be experienced
there is no shame in saying, "my time has come".
Mum, Joy, I hope this book honours your courage
your strength and your integrity in following your
truth.

Although this book is based on a true story, I have added, subtracted, adjusted, exaggerated, minimalised and just generally taken liberties with the all facts.
Enjoy! Laugh! Ponder! Discuss! Question!
But most of all have compassion.

Prologue

Have you ever wondered why animals are more advanced in the area of euthanasia?

How did they beat us superior humans past the post of empathy, logic, compassion and support?

Yes, it was a trick question! They didn't! It was we humans who decided it was acceptable to make an end of life decision for animals, based on life quality and longevity, i.e. compassion and common sense. Which must mean we either value our pets above ourselves, or we value them less?

Now from what I have seen and experienced when people make the decision to euthanize their pets, it is an heartbreaking experience and no less painful than if they were losing a family member, so I wouldn't be putting a tick in the box, "value them less".

(6th January 2014: 27 pilot whales were euthanized when they became beached on

Farewell Spit. *We carefully weighed up the likelihood of being able to refloat them and get them safely back out to sea which was not possible so rather than prolong their suffering we decided to euthanize them).*

So, why is it in most developed countries, the option for euthanasia is not available for the human species? Are we still facing the dilemma of being created by God in the "Garden of Eden" against the Darwinian theory of evolving over the millennia from apes?

The latter would mean it is ok to euthanize people, because basically we are just animals, admittedly some of us a bit more evolved than others. So, why hasn't it become an option for an end of life solution? Is it that God who loves us as his children, wants us to suffer? Wants us to keep experiencing pain, over and over and over? Hands up all those parents who want that for their children!

Could the answer be the former still holds a place in our psyches via guilt, punishment and shame?

Aren't they the most compassionate words you'll ever find in the dictionary? Words that have created more pain, sorrow and disempowerment than any others I could find.

Anyway, you're all kidding yourselves that it isn't happening. It is!

And that's what this book is about. About a normal person who has given herself the power to have choice. Choice over how she wants to live or die.

1

"Hello," I said, picking up the phone after a mad dash from the garden. Well I must admit it wasn't exactly a marathon! More like 5 metres really, but none the less a dash. My landline rarely went these days. Communications were texts or emails, so an actual phone call was quite unique and worthy of a dash.

"I've got it," the voice exclaimed, bubbling with excitement. It took me a few seconds to realise it was Mum. She never phoned me. Wasn't anything personal! She didn't phone anyone.

In her words, we all lived busy lives and she didn't want to intrude. This was partially the truth, but a more driven reason was the cost. International phone calls equated to dollar withdrawal and that's one addiction Mum was never going to suffer withdrawal from.

Mum came from a family of 10. She was the 5th child. Above her, 2 sisters and 2 brothers and following, 2 sisters and 3 brothers. If that wasn't reason enough to be frugal, it was exacerbated by the fact that her father was an alcoholic and they lived in a poor part of London in one of those 2 up, 2 down, council terraced houses, (like Coronation Street). Then when she was 8, there was World War 2 and evacuation. (Now there's another story) But to be brief, evacuation gave Mum an insight and strength that only those people who have been through adversity and come out the other side with their brain intact, can have.

Adversity can make or break you and as for that saying, *what doesn't kill you makes you stronger,* from my experience you don't need to go through a physical death to die. You can be dead inside but still walking the streets. Counselling for 10 years taught me that, as I saw some of the results of those things that *make you stronger!*

Anyway, quite a line-up really to make one appreciate the value of money. It was scarce. In Mum's mind it continued to be scarce. She was saving for World War 3. Admittedly not consciously, but the driving underlying thought was, *if I don't have money, I don't have choice* and choice was always important to Mum. Of course this was backed up by Dad's, *I would rather be miserable with money, than miserable without it.* He was a Scot, so say no more!

Not that Dad was there to reinforce Mum's already set in concrete lifestyle. He had been gone for 4 years. Irony played out at its best. Three years before Dad went, Mum had been diagnosed with breast cancer and had undergone a mastectomy, with a follow up of radiation treatment. No, they hadn't got IT. IT reappeared but didn't seem to be going anywhere in much of a hurry, which gave Dad the opportunity to get stomach and oesophageal cancer and beat Mum out of here. Now, I'm not a specialist, but... if you asked me, worry took Dad. Yes he was worried that if Mum went first, who would look after him? Who would cook his meals, do the washing, clean the house? Come to that, who would remind him to breath?

Yes, Mum was his lungs! The very reason he was alive and when those lungs looked like they were under the threat of collapse, he worried himself into oblivion.

"Best thing," Mum said, "that he went first. What the hell would he have done if I had gone and left him to it?" Not something anyone could even contemplate really! Mum was seventeen when they got engaged and eighteen when they married. Nearly made it to their sixtieth wedding anniversary, but... not quite.

Dad's mother died of TB when he was 3 and so when Mum came along, all full of common sense and drive, Dad handed over the mothering reins to her, which she picked up with gusto and continued to do so throughout their married life.

2

"Got what?" I asked, puzzled.

"You know, the stuff!"

"Ohhh!" I replied, as it dawned on me what she was talking about.

"But, they've only sent half of it!" I should have guessed, she sounded only half elated.

"Well that's great!" I replied sardonically. "What are you meant to do with that? Half kill yourself?"

"Hahaha, no," she splurted out, "they have split it into two shipments, so it wasn't such a bulky package. It arrived in a greeting card."

I laughed. "What did it say? Our sympathies on your impending bereavement?"

"No, it says, Bon Voyage. I hope your journey is full of excitement and adventure."

"Oh my God! Do you think they chose that on purpose or was it just coincidence? I wonder how good their English is?" Pause. "How do you feel now you're sort of halfway prepared?"

"Great! Like I've accomplished something really important. I hope the other half makes it through. Apparently they are checking all the Christmas mail thoroughly and there is a strong possibility of it being found."

"So what will you do then? Half is no good! This is not a journey you can do in halves!"

"Oh let's wait and see. They will probably wait until the holiday rush is over and send it after Christmas."

"Well, I guess you've no other choice but to do that! What does the stuff look like?"

"Like white powder, icing sugar."

"Oh, sweet!" I replied, my irony making me cringe. Part of me was happy for Mum because I knew she needed this choice, this preparation just in case. After nursing Dad through his cancer and watching him basically starve to death, she swore she wasn't going down the same path. So she set about gathering information on what her best options were.

Initially she came up with helium and got all the information on the pros and cons of exiting via this method. I never thought she would proceed with the helium option, although there were some very good specials of helium cylinders on sale at Spotlight Stores, which I thought might sway her into action. But even though the 50% discount was tempting, it wasn't tempting enough to get her over the image of lying on her bed with a plastic bag over her head.

So, while I went about my business preparing for the trip of a lifetime, 6 months in Europe, deciding a day at a time where I was going and what I'd do when I got there, Mum went about her business preparing for her trip of a lifetime, delving into the different modes of transport and the quickest and easiest way to get there.

Our lives often paralleled like this. Around the same time Dad died, the relationship I was in died also. We were now members of the same sisterhood, learning to re-establish ourselves as single women. For a while we were taking one step forward and two back, but the sharing about each other's experiences and the adventures and strengths we found in each other's journey, was the grease that kept the wheels turning.

3

"Hello," I said, putting the receiver to my ear wondering who the hell didn't know how to text or email in these days of electronic enlightenment.

"I've got it!" The voice screamed at me from across the Tasman Sea. It was early morning and I wondered if I was experiencing a case of déjà vu or another one of the lucid dreams I had experienced ever since I was a child.

No, I was awake! The reality check was sitting at my feet looking up at me with those expectant eyes of morning. Eyes that say, *you're my world, you're every breath I take. Now feed me.*

Oh God, it was too early to face the fact that my mother now had within her means the ability to take her own life. Up until that moment it had been like some sort of game.

It was called *Forbidden Fruit,* and went something like this. 250 points for locating the hiding place of the forbidden fruit. 250 further points if you can get the gold coins into the hiding place to open the lock to release each half of the forbidden fruit. 500 points per half, if you can then get the forbidden fruit past the dragons who guard it and the final whopping 5000 points if you manage to get both halves of the fruit to the magic chalice, which will turn the two halves into a whole and enable you to make the potion that turns you into a beautiful angel with translucent iridescent wings and an ability to live forever in the idyllic realms of the spirit world.

"Oh Mum that's wonderful!" I whispered, feeling torn between giving a lecture on not using it unless absolutely necessary and the doubtless knowledge that she wouldn't. One thing my Mum was not was a shrinking violet. She was not a quitter, but she was also realistic. I knew that if the time came, she would have thoroughly gone through all her options and make a decision based on objective logic.

"It must give you peace of mind," I empathised, "now you have choice. Even if you **never** use it, (emphasis on the never) you at least know you don't have to suffer like Dad did. That in itself was worth all the trouble of getting the stuff."

The stuff was Nembutal, bought from Asia with information gathered from Exit International. Mum was a ferret. She persisted until she found out where, how and what to do. Then she put it in her locked security cupboard, forgot about it and promptly got on with her life, living it her way and to her rhythm.

4

Mum was 82 and in good health apart from the cancer and arthritis which was particularly bad in her left foot. She often said the pain from the arthritis was worse than the cancer which she didn't find painful. This didn't work in her favour as I'll explain later.

Every morning as soon as the sun looked like it was going to pop its head over the horizon, she was off for her 8 kilometre walk to her local cafe where she would meet friends, exchange conversation with the staff and adopt those people who the rest of society would shun. There was Mathew who looked like an ex drug addict who would let his friends wheedle him out of his money and then not have enough for breakfast. He would often stand there having an incomprehensible conversation with himself and it was during these episodes Mum would ask him if he had taken his medication. She would also lend him the few dollars needed for a muffin and coffee and as soon as possible he would always pay her back.

Then there was Theresa, who was a transsexual. When Mum first met Theresa she hadn't been a woman for very long, having lived the first part of her 60 odd years as Ian. But when she finally decided to be honest with herself and her family as to how she truly felt, which was feminine, her family disowned her and she was left floundering as to how to transform herself from masculine into feminine in a way that the outside world would accept. Mum stepped in and adopted Theresa, but their interchange was only at the cafe. Mum's boundaries were firmly in place and her house and personal life were not up for grabs.

Theresa was told in no uncertain terms by Mum which clothes and wigs were acceptable for a woman of her age and physical build and slowly by the wave of Mum's magic wand, Theresa was transformed from a masculine looking woman in clothes that were a cross between a drag queen and the actual queen, to a trendy and soft looking woman.

There was also Sunshine, a gay guy Mum passed most days on her walk. They would say very little at first and mostly comment on the weather, until one day Sunshine looked more like a storm cloud than the happy guy she exchanged pleasantries with. "Whatever's the matter?" she exclaimed when she saw his forlorn look. He told her he had lost someone close to him and because she had recently lost Dad, they bonded and shared their journey of grief together. Amazing what a difference a stranger can make in a few minutes of interchange when passing each other on their morning journey.

Mum's table at the café was like a counselling booth with the comings and goings of people who wanted to get some truth and advice about their lives. Occasionally Sunshine would bump into Mum at the café and give her a big hug.

Mum's aptitude for empathy and style was reinforced when Theresa once commented that Mum's advice had never let her down and had always enhanced her life.

And Mathew who a month after Mum's passing, was still talking about, "you know Joy, the lady who used to sit over there, who died. I miss her. I still owe her money."

These were people who needed people and Mum was the person who would shoot from the hip and tell them the truths that no one else would. Honesty was her gift to them.

Prior to leaving for this important ritual of her day, Mum would text my sister and me to reassure us she was still alive and kicking, but normally it took the form of a weather report and went something like... *sun's shining, wind's blowing and I'm off*. Or, *sun's up, I'm off before it gets too hot*. Ever since she had had the radiation, Mum couldn't cope with heat and was very conscious of the sun's effect on her physical body. I would reply in like, *raining here, just for a change, need to take Griffy for his walk but too wet*. Or *raining and windy here Griffy doesn't want to get his feet wet*! Griffy was my Dog. A Cavoodle. Yes the one who every morning looks at me with those big innocent manipulative eyes, that say, "yes, without me you'd be experiencing empty nest syndrome big time! You owe me!"

Mum had also pre-warned us that if she was going to take "the stuff" she would send a special text. The text would say, *gone to see Dad*. Just that! Nothing more elaborate. No phone calls to say, so long it's been good to know you! That wasn't her style.

She hated goodbyes and would avoid them at all costs. Inside she was putty, outside she was concrete. There were only a few people who had the required formula to get through to the putty and even then the airing of the putty was brief. Probably didn't want to get it sunburnt so she made sure it was kept covered and in the shade.

5

So, with the security of the "stuff" in her cupboard, Mum got on with her life and I went off overseas to experience what true freedom was. No deadlines, no have tos, no answering to, just "what do I want to do with this day?" It was liberating, relaxing, informative, challenging and above all I learnt to trust in life and my intuition. If it said head to Paris, I would head to Paris and there in an apartment in the centre of Paris I drowned myself in French culture.

If it said go to Greece, I went to Greece or at least Kefalonia, a Greek Island off the coast of the mainland, and stayed for a month in a villa up the road from an exquisite local beach, whose waters were turquoise and surrounding cliffs white. The couple who owned the villa adopted me and I became part of their family and enjoyed some wonderful cooking lessons with Maria, gathering most of the ingredients straight out of her garden. She couldn't speak English and I couldn't speak Greek, so in a hilarious recipe of pigeon English, pigeon Greek and pigeon sign language, we muddled on through. When we hit a barrier and just couldn't surmount it with all the pigeon, we would throw our hands up in the air and burst out laughing. By the time her husband Nikos came home and started filling me in on all the local history, Maria had pretty much been there and done that. He looked completely puzzled as he knew our communication barrier was well and truly in place, but he hadn't allowed for the wonderful bond we shared, the mutual love of laughing and the unusual sign language we developed.

They invited me to the Island's traditional music and dancing night, which was followed a couple of weeks later with the Midsummer solstice ritual. This was the night when the locals all got together at a neighbourhood school and built a bonfire. Once it was lit and the flames were dancing out the top, the kids started to jump over it. I was just about to go and save them, when an elderly woman came along and proceeded to line herself up and then take a flying leap over the fire also. At this point I figured there must be an ulterior motive for singeing and smoking one's nether regions, so I rushed off to have my suspicions confirmed by Nikos who informed me, it was the solstice ritual of cleansing and purification. He asked if I would like to try and jump the fire but I declined, explaining I had had two swims that day and a shower after each, so felt I was as cleansed and purified as I was ever going to be. Besides I didn't fancy inhaling smoke, either up my nether regions or through my nose or mouth. He laughed when I came back with I hadn't seen him do it yet.

My next adventure was in a small English village where I stayed in an old thatched weaver's cottage, owned by a wonderful woman called Helen. The first night I was there, the village had a New Zealand wine tasting evening and I was invited along as the Kiwi Nation's representative. It was so much fun and not being much of a drinker, I was well on my way after the first few samples (no I never saw anyone spit it out) and the hilarity of the differing opinions when we had to fill out the tasting forms made me realise that taste is very much a personal thing and in particular when you are that tipsy, you don't really care.

The next night the village had a musical evening and because I was now part of the thatching, I was invited along to join in the merriment. The music was superb and the singing sublime. There was a guy playing a fiddle who added a dimension to some of the music, which surpassed the ordinary. It brought tears to my eyes and touched my soul.

As I left everyone was asking me which house I was going to buy, as I had been absorbed so quickly into this wonderful, supportive environment. An environment which is seldom experienced in today's impersonal hectic suburban lifestyle.

I visited Wales and stayed with a couple who were old hippies from the 60s. Yes, they had done the whole 'make love not war' demonstrations, smoked pot and lived in a commune. They were still very much into getting back to the land and nurtured their beliefs in their small land holding which they farmed with much enthusiasm.

I'll never forget driving out of their driveway on my way to another adventure and my car being scattered with flowers and petals as I passed and waved goodbye to two of the kindest and chilled out people I have ever met.

During all of these and many more adventures I would keep Mum up to date with regular epistle like texts and scattered phone calls with which she would always affirm, *keep up the texts I feel like I am on the journey with you.*

6

One day, later in my journey, I phoned Mum to see how she was going and catch her up on my latest adventures. I hardly got a word in when she blurted out, "I've got something to tell you."

Oh dear, I thought, "what's happened?"

"You know those coughing fits I've been having, well they're getting worse and sometimes I can't get my breath because all this mucus builds up at the back of my throat and I choke. I had one on the bus the other day, just before my stop and the driver couldn't get me off the bus quick enough. I'm sure he thought I was going to choke to death on his bus. He took off at such a speed as soon as I was off. I would have burst out laughing if I could have got a breath."

"Anyway that's all beside the point. I need to tell you what happened the other night. You know how you have all those visions and dreams and people talking to you in your sleep and I've always wished I had had some experiences like that, because I'm such a doubter and don't believe a thing unless it happens to me. Well the other night I took a sleeping pill to help me sleep as I haven't been sleeping all that well lately and after taking the pill, I must have drifted off into a very deep sleep, because you came and visited me and said to me, "Mum wake up, Mum wake up, Mum wake up". Just like that. Three times in a normal voice, no yelling, no screaming, and you were standing there beside my bed clear as day. Well after the third, "Mum wake up", I came to and realised I wasn't breathing as the phlegm had lodged itself at the back of my throat and blocked off my windpipe. If you hadn't come and told me to wake up, I would have died as I was in such a deep sleep I was totally unaware of what was going on. Isn't that amazing! I know what you're talking about now! It's as though you're awake, the experience is as real as daytime."

"That's great Mum, at least now you know there's more to life than what you see when you're awake and thank goodness you're ok."

"Isn't it amazing?" she continued, not the slightest bit interested in the fact that she nearly suffocated to death. "To think you can see

23

another side like that! Oh I'm so pleased I had that experience."

Esoteric experiences were not new to me. As a child I saw spirits floating around my room, which to be honest scared the living daylights out of me, to the extent I used to get out of bed and stand beside Mum for security and comfort while she was asleep.

One night I was standing there getting my dose of security, when she awoke and just about had a heart attack. "For Christ's sake Diane," she said, "you scared the living daylights out of me."

I never told her the things floating around in my room were doing the same to me.

After a while I stopped seeing them, but continued to have lucid dreams. Dreams where colours are so vibrant everything else pales in comparison. And voices who teach and sing, and scenarios that depict some part of my life, whether past, present or future. Once I heard the most exquisite women's choir singing a very poignant song. The words were about women who had found themselves on their own, through war, death, separation etc. and who had found their own strength through their loss. It was like they were welcoming me into their fold as I was experiencing my first journey into life as a single woman. A life where I was responsible for making all the decisions and there was no safety net to catch me if I fell.

It was magical, reassuring, haunting and I awoke crying.

"Mum I think you should go and see the doctor and find out what's happening in your throat."

Mum's cancer which had never really disappeared, but just kept everyone guessing as to where it was going to pop up next, eventually decided to settle in the cavity between the lungs with more of a leaning towards the heart and upper chest and throat area. You could actually see the mass and notice the increase in size as it travelled slowly from left to right heading upwards towards her throat like a snake under the skin.

Mum had already undergone intensive radiotherapy and there were only so many doses she could have. When the cancer returned the doctors told Mum to wait until the cancer was at a point where it was worth using the remaining doses and when she told them, "it doesn't hurt and is not interfering with my life in anyway," she more or less took the seriousness and urgency out of the situation which put her in a position of wait and see. I guess because she was still walking 8ks every day it didn't seem to be that dire.

At that point in Mum's medical conundrum her doctor was desperately trying to get her red blood cell count in order as it was low and she couldn't figure out why. She put Mum on blood thickeners, medication that would increase her cell count, and booked Mum in for a colonoscopy and esophagoscopy.

"What can she do? She already has me booked in for those tests which will tell her what's going on. I'll wait for those, they can't be that far away."

"I don't know Mum, this seems more urgent than sitting around waiting for something that could be months off!"

"No, I think I'll wait."

"Ok!" I replied unconvinced. I would have pushed harder for her to follow up with her doctor but once Mum had made her mind up to do something there was no turning her around unless you had cold hard facts to persuade her otherwise. Also, in a few weeks I would be with her. I had organised a 2 week stopover in Australia on my way back to NZ, to be with her for her 82nd birthday.

7

Mum's exploration into Euthanasia was no secret. She told everyone. Her favourite line was, "no way am I going to be sitting in a home, dribbling over my meal, waiting to be force fed because the only way I can get out of there is to starve myself to death." She would also affirm to everyone that they were on her list to be notified when she had gone.

Everyone knew she attended the Exit International meetings and she would share with them all the information gathered. She often affirmed that when she couldn't do her morning walk, it was going to be time to re-evaluate.

I don't know if any of us who knew Mum and her investigations into euthanasia actually believed she would do it. I looked at it more as a safeguard against the nightmarish slow death my father experienced, but because of Mum's strong constitution, actually thought she would die of a heart attack or stroke doing that morning walk, rather than experience a long lingering death.

The words "long & lingering" didn't fit Mum. She was more "short and sweet". Or, maybe even, "short and sharp". She didn't waste time thinking about things, she was an action lady. Make a decision and do it! And then if it hit the fan after that, re-evaluate and then do something about that too.

When Dad died and we organised his funeral, Mum started thinking about her own. Not one to sit and ponder on things for too long, she marched off down the highway to the funeral home and organised and paid for her own funeral. She chose her coffin, the celebrant and then informed me what songs and readings she wanted included in the ceremony.

"Great," she said to me, "I can cross that one off the list." She was relieved! It was one less thing to think about.

"Now all you need to do is make a phone call and the Funeral Director will take it from there. Here are their contact details," she dictated through the phone.

Mum lived on her own in Australia. My sister and I lived in NZ and Mum's siblings were in the UK. Mum and Dad decided to retire in Australia because of the weather. They called retirement and their life in Australia, *a permanent holiday.*

The warmer drier weather was kinder to Mum's arthritis, whereas Auckland's weather being cold and damp seemed to torture, torment, inflame and irritate arthritis.

The morning weather forecast texts were a testimony to this.

Sunny again, she would text.

Raining again, I would reply.

8

Before heading off to Australia I spent some time with Mum's family down in Portsmouth. I hadn't seen most of them for 55 years and some of them I had never met at all. I was four when Mum and Dad emigrated to NZ and really can't remember anything about my life prior to that.

My son and granddaughter came down from London and met all their English relatives for the first time and it was amazing to see the family resemblances. My son was the spitting image of Mum's youngest brother, to the extent when the photos came out people were confusing them for each other.

I also discovered when chatting with my Auntie that she and Nana both had psychic experiences. I always wondered where it came from but had no point of reference to find out. Funnily enough knowing this gave me peace of mind. I guess I always thought I was kind of bonkers and wondered why no one else could see what I saw.

Being bonkers in a group is much more acceptable than bonkers on your own.

Mum's brothers and sisters were all worried about her and the cancer but being on the other side of the world, were too far away to do anything to help apart from the phone calls they made over the weekends, and which I am sure if my calls were anything to go by, Mum hogged all the airtime. She informed them about her euthanasia plans also. Why not? She had told everyone else. It was like she was warning them, preparing them, so that when they got the call she had gone, it wouldn't be so much of a shock.

They were all reassured when I informed them I was going to stay with Mum for a couple of weeks prior to going home to celebrate her birthday with her and see just what sort of state she was in.

I left my relatives feeling like I had reconnected with my roots and had a newfound sense of family, after a lifetime of floundering around not knowing where I fit.

After saying goodbye to everyone I jumped on the train to Heathrow, lugging two overfull suitcases wondering how the hell I would manage to get them safely home. I still had to get them to Mum's and then back to the airport and on the plane to NZ.

My family in NZ were going to meet me off the plane so once there it was not a problem, but prior to that I had buses and 5 flights of stairs to surmount to get to Mum's apartment.

9

My flight was uneventful and I managed a slight snooze, but am not one of those people you see snoring their heads off for most of the journey. I try and lessen the impact by watching movies and eating and grin and bear the rest.

I arrived at Coolangatta airport around 7:30pm and by the time I got the shuttle and made it up the 5 flight of stairs, I fell through Mum's apartment door around 10:30pm.

I had keys so she didn't need to wait up for me. Mum was an early to bed person and that usually meant she was asleep shortly after 7:30pm. But in saying that she was also an early to rise person, anytime from 3 to 4am. By the time the sun was up, Mum was already pounding the footpath and sometimes in summer that was 4:30am.

"Hello stranger!" this voice said, from somewhere in the darkened room. Her greeting took me by surprise!

"What are you still doing up?" I gasped, sounding like a smoker of 50 years or a person having a severe asthma attack. It wasn't so much the stairs but the suitcases I had to lug up them that had me gulping for air. My eyes were still adjusting to the dimness when Mum turned the light on and my eyes had to adjust back to where they were moments before.

Mum often sat in the dark looking out over the street. She lived opposite a large apartment block which had restaurants and retail outlets underneath. She and Dad moved in to their apartment when there was very little around them, or at least only 2 level buildings.

Slowly the older blocks were purchased and up went buildings that continued to beat each other in their monstrositiness and theirs which was once one of the better apartment blocks, ended up being an ok apartment block squeezed between phallic symbols of all shapes, sizes and colours.

Objectively, this wasn't a bad progression in development, as it gave Mum something to watch and interact with while it was going on. She got to know the building site managers on a first name basis and could often be found without her hard hat on, discussing the best place to position the swimming pool, or what sort of trees would be beneficial in a certain area.

She even helped out by phoning the council and letting them know the glare from the sun reflecting off the windows in the new development opposite would heat up her place to an unhealthy degree and suggested a good design feature to counteract this would be external louvers. Yes the building now has external louvers and Mum doesn't have to sit and fret over the potential possibility of reflected heat. Mind you, I think the people who work in the office where the windows are, appreciate the filtered light more than Mum.

Mum was the caretaker of all that came within her vicinity and didn't worry too much about repercussions, just justice and what was fair.

One night she must have been prowling around her apartment in the dark when she heard some guys off the street, jumping over the wall and diving into the swimming pool which was directly under her balcony. Without hesitation she opened her ranch slider and told them to "bugger off." When they answered back she showed them the phone in her hands and informed them, the cops who were one block down the road, were on their way. They laughed, jumped out of the pool and hurdled back across the wall yelling at the top of their voices, "we've just been told off by a golden oldie." She thought it was hilarious, as were the several naked young men who would end up taking midnight skinny dips in the pool on their way home from the night clubs.

Mum didn't believe in backing down, if something wasn't fair. She'd fight tooth and nail for justice, not just for herself but for others also. Once she got on a full bus and there were teenagers sitting in the seats that were prioritised for pensioners, the disabled or people with prams. They didn't move a muscle, so Mum stood over them and said, "hey you two, up!" "Well," she said, "they couldn't get up quick enough." That was my Mum.

"No point in going to bed, I wouldn't have slept anyway!"

"You're looking good," I told her as I gave her a big hug. "I expected to find you half dead with that cough you've got."

"Yes, don't I," she agreed. "Unfortunately that's the medication the doctors have me on to increase my blood count. It makes me retain fluid and because of that my face has swollen and made all the wrinkles disappear."

"What a shame! It suits you."

We spent the next hour having a catch up on everything and nothing and I crawled into bed around midnight.

10

I slept 12 hours that night and when I did eventually emerge from my cocoon, Mum had already been for her walk, had breakfast and lunch and was contemplating what to have for dinner.

I discovered when staying with them years before, the big decisions of the day when you're retired are what to eat for your meals. These discussions could go on for hours. In fact it was a good thing they did or the days would have seemed indeterminably long.

I stood at my bedroom door looking at Mum sitting there in her chair watching the world go by and I was surprised to see she wasn't knitting. Mum had been knitting since she was 8 and over the past few years had knitted beautiful baby shawls which she sent to me in NZ and I sold on her behalf on eBay. Those shawls ended up all over the world, from London to New York, and the comments were always full of gratitude.

Please thank your mother for this beautiful shawl. She is so clever and we are thrilled with it. I couldn't be happier with the shawl, it is amazing, please pass on our thanks to your Mum and tell her we love it.

It was a poignant moment, one of those moments when you realise this was the woman who gave birth to you, who fed and clothed you and gave you everything she couldn't have even imagined herself getting as a child.

"Good afternoon," she said with emphasis on the afternoon. "I was going to give you another hour and then check to see if you were still alive!"

"Yeah!" I replied, "I have serious jetlag, I feel a bit dizzy. I'm going to make a cuppa, do you want one?"

"Yes please!"

I was brought up on tea. I think I may even have had it in my feeding bottle. I know some nights when Mum and Dad had their evening cuppa, Dad would sneak down the hall and see if my sister and I were awake and if we were he would bring us one in bed. A cuppa is the first thing I turn to when the going gets tough.

I put Mum's cup down on the table beside her chair. It was her, "I don't have to get up for anything table", because "everything but the kitchen sink" is here. Nail files, Vaseline, band aids, scissors, phone, notebook, address book, pens, magazines, glasses, etc.

I dropped into the chair next to hers. It used to be Dad's chair but since he had vacated it, it was permanently facing into the room, while Mum's chair was permanently facing the street.

Mum would alternate between the chairs, if there was a programme on the TV she wanted to watch she would sit in Dad's chair, if not, she would always be in the other, watching the world go by.

"Not knitting?" I enquired, trying to sound nonchalant. Mum was sharp as tacks and didn't miss a trick. Not only did she experience things during evacuation that no child should go through, but she had worked as a clerk in a locked ward in a psychiatric hospital. So what senses she hadn't honed as a child, she sharpened in the hospital.

"No, haven't really felt like it lately. Weather must be getting too hot!"

"Oh! Is there anything you want to do today, or what's left of it?" I ventured, changing the subject to get the blood hound off my trail.

"We could go to Pacific Fair, I need to get some avocados and they're cheaper there."

"Great," I replied enthusiastically. I figured I could drag myself across to Pacific Fair before I collapsed into another jetlag coma. "What time shall we head off?"

"After you've had something to eat, then we can be back in time to watch *Last of the Summer Wine* on TV."

"Sounds like a plan," I agreed heading off to the kitchen to get some food.

11

The first few days went by like this. Me sleeping or trying not to, followed by our trips to various shopping centres to stock up on essentials.

Mum's cough wasn't good. It was always there! Sometimes just a small episode or a clearing of the throat and then other times a good old hack.

While I was there over the two week period I never saw Mum have a coughing episode where she couldn't get her breath, but there were occasions when I thought *something's not right* and said so.

"Mum, I'm not happy about that cough of yours. I think you should go to the doctors."

"I've already been and that is one of the reasons I am having the oesophageal test. I can't do anything more because they need that test to see what's going on!"

"Well, when is that going to happen? Do they know how urgent it is? I think I should phone the doctor and have a chat with her about everything. What do you think?"

"Diane, you can do what you want, but I'll still have to wait for the test."

Shit! I thought. *What do I do?* I had already upset Mum when I asked her when she had last vacuumed. There was fluff all over the carpet which was very unusual for her. Mum was always spotless to the point of being anal.

"I don't care," she informed me defiantly. "I just don't care. I'll do it when I feel like it."

Oh God! I didn't like what I was seeing. No knitting, housework gone to the dogs. Eating was only undertaken because she knew if she didn't she wouldn't have the energy to be able to get out for her walk.

And then there were the visits. Visits to places where she and Dad used to go. They were always at her suggestion.

"What would you like to do today?" I would ask through a fog of Jetlag that seemed to go on forever.

"Let's go to Twin Towns," she suggested. Which was where Mum and Dad used to go dancing, or *Australia Fair* or *Robina,* which was where they used to alternate their shopping excursions.

It really didn't hit me until I surprised Mum with a birthday seafood lunch in a revolving restaurant where the views were magnificent and you could see right along the coast and back to the hinterland. It was an over view of her stomping ground.

The revolution took an hour and it was during this hour that it dawned on me. Mum was saying goodbye. Goodbye to all the places that meant something to her. Goodbye to all her old haunts. The places where she and Dad had spent time having fun or where she had wandered on her own to have her time.

Oh hell, I thought, and once again, *what do I do*?

Nothing, said a voice in my head.

Nothing! I exclaimed.

Yes! Nothing! This is her journey. Your job is to keep her company. She is preparing.

Oh shit, oh shit, oh shit! I thought, looking at her and holding back the tears.

"More prawns?" I asked, trying to escape to the buffet to collect myself.

"Oh yes please, these are delicious. What a wonderful birthday I'm having!"

I just about knocked my chair over trying to get to the prawns and escape before the tears gave me away.

12

From then on, for me it was different. I got up in the morning, no matter what ungodly hour and walked the 8k to Surfers and back. I went with Mum to wherever she suggested and watched her face as she looked at what had been a major part of her life.

If the floor was fluffy I vacuumed and didn't say anything. If the toilet and bathroom needed cleaning I got on with it. I lived a life around Mum's life, that was conscious and knowing. While she went about her daily business, following some sort of inner guidance that was helping her say goodbye.

The question was always, when?

I would get up in the morning, half expecting to see her bedroom door still shut, but no, every morning she was there sitting in her chair, watching the early regulars head off to work and checking her clock to make sure they were on time.

Phew! I would think and continue on to appreciate whatever the day brought.

"He's late this morning," she would declare if there were a few minutes discrepancy when he appeared.

"Oh, she's parked there. She never normally parks there. I wonder why." Mum loved a good mystery, a good, *Who Dunnit.* She usually had picked the culprit a few minutes into the programme.

"Oh really! Him? Are you sure?" I would say, knowing damned well she would be right and it was just a matter now of seeing how the script writers filled in the blanks.

So, on we went through our parallel journey. Me in the 'www' world of wondering, watching, waiting and Mum going about her business of saying goodbye and totally oblivious to the fact that she was doing so.

This is how we spent our last days together, until it was time for me to head back to NZ and pick up the pieces of my life, which I had abandoned 6 months previously.

Realistically I couldn't stay just because my intuition said Mum's getting ready to go. I had to go and pick up my life, I had to find a job and collect my dog from the angel who had looked after him while I gallivanted off overseas. So, with the reassuring knowledge my sister was going to arrive in a few days to spend time with Mum, I headed off back to NZ to pick up the pieces of a life I now realised I wanted to change in quite a few ways.

It was early but not any earlier than Mum's morning walk, when I took my suitcases to the top of the first flight of stairs. I stood there looking down, wondering how they would cope if I just gave them a little nudge, so they would slide easefully down the stairs without any injuries to my arms or back, but thought better of it when I remembered there was someone on the next level probably still fast asleep. So I slowly made my way down the 4 flights (didn't need to go through the basement, so luckily it was one flight less than when I arrived) with each bag and out onto the footpath to wait for the bus.

To my surprise Mum stood with me to wait for the shuttle. But admittedly she was ready to sprint off on her morning walk the minute I was on the bus, so she could hide the tears.

We both saw the shuttle coming down the road and hugged in anticipation of our separation. She didn't cry until she was off down the road and I didn't cry until the shuttle drove passed her and I saw her tears.

Oh shit, oh shit, oh shit, I thought! *There's nothing I can do*!

13

For most of my flight home I sat looking out the window trying to think of something I could do to solve my dilemma.

How would, *Mum you're going to die soon, trust me I know,* work out?

Or, *Mum, you know how sometimes I know things before they happen, well you're showing all the signs of someone saying goodbye to life.*

But what difference would it make even if she believed me? What would it change? I knew for a fact she wouldn't come back to NZ. She would lose all she had worked so hard to attain, her freedom and independence.

Ignorance is bliss, I thought, I wish I didn't know. So leave Mum in her bliss and pray that I am wrong. So, that's how I proceeded on with my life, knowing that Mum was proceeding on with hers, oblivious to my concerns.

I walked out of customs and through the exit looking at the maze of people standing waiting. Then I spotted them. My wonderful, caring, beautiful daughters-in-law and my four delicious grand-children. My grandchildren were holding a banner, saying, "Welcome Home" on it. They had all grown taller and knew more words than when I left. The two two-year-olds had learnt the word, "no", which they exercised with much authority, while the other two, one four and one three-year-old had bonded and become the best of friends.

I had hoped by taking my overseas trip at this time in my life and my families' lives that I would come home and not find too much changed. This had been the case and I slotted back into my role as Nana, Mum and Mother-in-law very quickly.

My sons and daughter-in-laws had a welcome home barbecue for me and it was a joy to see all the children playing together as only close cousins can.

I collected Griffy once I had unpacked, worrying he wouldn't remember who the hell I was. But there was no chance of that and the minute he saw me, he went into his meet and greet frantic routine, where he talks to you by making grunting sounds from the back of his throat. He was probably saying, *where the hell have you been all this time? Don't you know you promised to love, honour and obey me?* Once he had forgiven me, I took him home and watched him go about his usual business as though he had never been away.

After my sister had visited Mum and returned to NZ, I went back to my old routine of phoning Mum most evenings. She seemed in good form and apart from the cough, which occasionally interrupted her monologue, her life was progressing much as usual.

I applied for a few jobs and succeeded in getting one which started in the New Year, so got on about my business reconnecting with family and friends. I had been home 2 weeks.

14

I can't remember what I was doing when I got the phone call, I know I was at home but it is all a bit of a blur. I could hardly hear the voice on the other end of the phone, it was very faint and what I could hear was croaky.

I worked out it was Mum from her London accent, she was on her way to hospital. She had had another one of those coughing fits, but this one was serious and she had visited her doctor who ordered an immediate scan and a few hours after that she was on her way to hospital in an ambulance, having been diagnosed with a blood clot in her throat which was choking off her windpipe.

The blood thickeners she was on to increase her blood count were dropped like hot bricks and blood thinners were introduced by the quickest means possible via a drip. "I'll be all right," she assured me.

"Like hell," I said ignoring her and moving towards the computer to book a flight back to Australia. "I'll let you know when my flight arrives." After finding out where they were taking her, I hung up and immediately phoned her doctor to get the prognosis from the horse's mouth. That way I could make a more informed decision, rather than basing it on the information Mum had given me which was always understated to say the least.

Her doctor gave me a brief run down on the problems Mum was facing and finished by saying, "yes, I think it would be a good idea if you came over to support her. Your mother is a very strong woman and handles things in a stoic way, but in this case I think it would be nice for her to have family here."

I phoned my sister to discuss what her plans were and because she had used up all her leave visiting her daughter in Brisbane and Mum afterwards, it was a practical decision for me to go. I booked the flight and then a shuttle to take me straight to the hospital and then phoned my sister back to let her know.

15

I found Mum sitting in a chair in the ward TV room looking out at the bustling street below, watching people go about their business. Nothing had changed! She had just swapped one vantage point for another and continued on with her favourite past time of watching the world go by.

"Hello love", she croaked! "I was looking out to see if I could see you arrive, but you must have come a different way."

She looked paler than when I had seen her a few weeks earlier. "How's it going?" I enquired.

"Oh not bad, apart from that woman in the bed next to me who won't shut up. I'm managing!"

"Do you know she was talking to one of the nurses at two in the morning? Not just whispering but talking and laughing as though it was middle of the day! I ask you. I had to tell them I was trying to sleep and to be quiet."

Lois, the woman in the bed next to Mum, wasn't in good shape. She had bone cancer and a few cracked vertebrae, so when she moved she was in agony and grunted and groaned her way to and from the shared toilet. She was blocked up and although she was doing her utmost, (from the sounds of it), to make things happen. Her agonising marathons, well more like a 5 metre dash really, at a snail's pace, to the releasing chamber, were a waste (pardon the pun) of time.

Medication and food were being ingested at a rate of knots to try to induce delivery and after several false starts, there was a blessed release. Lois came out smiling but apologetic and quickly went off to announce to the world a weight had been lifted off her shoulders. She returned pushing her walker in front of her enabling her to alternately slide each foot in the direction she was heading. Behind her in convoy was a line of inspectors and eventually last but by no means least, the cleaner, who like a true Aussie Digger with a smile on her face, went over the top and confronted the enemy.

Now my mother, who watched this whole process take place, rolled her eyes and informed me, she was getting out of there as quickly as possible.

The good thing about her admittance into hospital was the tests they had undertaken while she was there. They left no stone unturned and by the time Mum left hospital the following day, she had discovered, she had gall stones, a hernia, arthritis throughout her body and the cancer which had now taken over her chest cavity to the extent it was pushing all her organs around in places they weren't meant to be and hence created the blood clot that was blocking off her windpipe.

In a couple of days she walked out of hospital with a truck load of syringes with which she was to inject herself twice a day to thin her blood. Obviously the thickening of the blood had become less of a priority than the cutting off of her windpipe, so in a 180 manoeuvre that any rally driver would be proud of, blood thinners became the driving force in keeping Mum alive.

Her abdomen which was where she injected herself twice daily looked like she had participated in a paintball war and her stomach was the bull's eye to practice on.

I could almost time the effect the injection had on Mum. Within 10 minutes of having the blood thinners, she was asleep. They made her feel dizzy, weak and lethargic. The worst result from them was Mum couldn't do her walk. She had no energy and would often say before the injection, "Let's go for our walk this morning. I'm feeling ok."

"Shall we see how you feel after you've had your injection, you know how it affects you," I'd suggest, feeling like I had just taken a lolly off a child.

One morning Mum suggested she do her walk before she had the injection that way she could still get out and about, so I accompanied her on her journey to her favourite café. She made it there ok, but on the way home I could tell she was struggling.

I think she was testing herself to see if the walk was still possible because since she had been injecting the blood thinners, her life had seemed to come to almost a standstill. After a while she realised the walk was just too much of a struggle and when I suggested she do a smaller one, she said it wouldn't be the same.

She also left the hospital with an appointment to meet with the Oncologist and prior to that two other appointments. One for an ultrasound and the other for a CT scan at nuclear medicine, where she was to be injected with radioactive dye so the affected areas would show up.

Mum insisted we caught the bus to and from the hospital, she wasn't going to pay for a taxi when the results were the same. Both stops were outside the hospital's main entrance and the bus stop by her apartment was not even a block away.

We arrived home and I put the kettle on. Mum looked a bit tired, so I suggested she have a rest while I prepare some lunch. "I'm not tired," she informed me, but sat down anyway and was asleep before I'd made the tea.

Mum's naps were never for very long, maybe 5 to 10 minutes at the most, and she always awoke refreshed as if she had been asleep for hours.

We discussed the upcoming appointments and I put them in my iPhone calendar to remind me in plenty of time to get ready. We both agreed the scan and ultrasound were to check exactly how far the cancer had travelled, whether it had spread into any vital organs and from there would come the decision as to what treatment would follow.

The ultrasound was very quick but the CT scan took longer than anticipated, so I found a seat in the corner of the hospital café and caught up on all the latest Hollywood gossip from some of the magazines that were floating around. When I went back to get Mum from the CT scan I was told I was not to be any closer to Mum than approximately one and a half metres as she was giving off radiation. I wondered if we were in the dark, whether she would glow and when I did get too close I had a metallic taste on the back of my tongue, so God knows what it was doing to Mum's insides.

True to form Mum insisted we take the bus home, so I'm not sure who got irradiated and who didn't. I don't know if they think about things like that when they inject people with radioactive material. Not everyone can afford a taxi and not everyone has someone around who drives.

I know there are drivers who take cancer patients to and from the hospital when they have chemotherapy, but Mum wasn't in the system yet, so although I did enquire, that was not an option.

16

Today was the day! The appointment with the oncologist was looming and Mum would find out the results of all her tests and see what her options were in regards to the treatment.

We caught the bus to the hospital as usual and went to the cancer clinic to register with the reception there.

Initially a nurse called Mum to take some details and check her weight and then she returned to the general waiting area to wait for the oncologist.

The room was full. There were people in wheel chairs, people with no hair, people with scarves on their heads, people with hats and people with hair which was obviously growing back after having fallen out.

They were all ages, but Mum was by far the oldest and they all had one thing in common, a hollow look in their eyes. A look that said they knew what pain and suffering were.

Mum's name was called and this time I accompanied her to see the oncologist. I wanted to hear what he had to say and ask questions if I felt there was something not mentioned or was overlooked. Mum was notorious for talking over the top of people and in the end a lot of information was lost because of her interruptions.

The first thing he explained to Mum was exactly where the cancer had spread. It had taken over the chest cavity and as a result the organs were being pushed up because of lack of space. This information was nothing new and had already been diagnosed when the blood clot had been discovered. What was new was that it was heading towards the heart and lungs and had reached up near the larynx and oesophagus.

The radiation treatment Mum had always thought was her safety net was not an option now as she didn't have enough doses left for it to be effective, so the Oncologist informed Mum the best and only option was to have chemotherapy.

He asked her how she felt about that and Mum came back very quickly with, "I don't want it."

Now I don't know why and I have looked back in my memory several times to go over those moments when Mum told him she didn't want chemotherapy but it seemed to be a blip in the flow of conversation that was completely overlooked and the conversation continued on as if she had never uttered those four words.

He didn't stop and I didn't stop but we continued on talking about the programme that would be put in place for Mum, in regards to how often and what to expect.

"There are several types of chemo available and some of the affects you may experience are, hair loss, nausea/vomiting, diarrhoea/constipation, mouth/gum/throat problems, sensitive dry skin, fever, tiredness and headaches to mention a few. Now nothing's set in concrete, because everyone reacts differently, but these are potential side effects.

"Also because the chemotherapy attacks both the good and diseased cells in the body, you will be prone to infections, so you should stay away from anyone who has a cold or anything that is contagious because your immune system will be at an all-time low. If you get a cold, then it is highly likely it will develop into pneumonia."

I sat there looking at this 82 year old woman who was just told she was going to be tortured and tried to gauge her reaction, there was nothing. Her face was a blank slate.

"Can you tell me what the prognosis is for Mum when she has completed the chemotherapy treatment?"

"Well it won't cure it! That chance has passed and is only available with the initial treatments when the cancer is first discovered. Once secondaries have set in, we're looking at holding it at bay to extend life and improve life quality!

"Of course the chemo might not work at all. There really are no guarantees, but we can always try something else if our first choice doesn't work!"

"Sorry! Can I reiterate what you've just said so I am sure I've got it correct? Mum will always have cancer because it wasn't eradicated with the initial treatment. What the chemo will do is hold it at bay, to give Mum the possibility of a longer life and a life that may improve in quality?"

"Yes! That's correct."

Mum was still sitting there looking like stone.

"So when does the treatment begin?"

"Well we could start it next week if you want?"

"Mum is that ok with you?" I enquired, to try and bring her back into the room and participate in what was to be her future.

"Yes," she said from someplace far away.

"Ok," said the oncologist, "I'll get the nurse to set up the appointments and introduce you to your support person."

The nurse then took us to a room in another corridor where a lovely woman came in and introduced herself to Mum as her support person. The person Mum was to contact for everything and anything.

She took all Mum's details and asked her a lot of questions. It was my turn to sit there like stone and take in what had just happened. In that moment I made a decision, a decision that from this point forward, I would have no opinion. I would walk beside Mum and keep her company. I would listen to what she had to say, but everything had to be Mum's decision. This was important, because I knew she had the "stuff" sitting in her security cupboard at home and I was not going to influence in any way what my mother wanted her future to be. I couldn't. It was not my life, Mum had all her faculties, she knew what she wanted her life to be and what she could and couldn't handle.

Words started echoing in my head. The words I heard when we were celebrating Mum's 82nd birthday in the revolving restaurant. Words that said;

Oh hell, what do I do?

Nothing!

Nothing?

Yes! Nothing! This is her journey. Your job is to keep her company. She is preparing.

Oh shit, oh shit, oh shit!

Now, in the support person's office, I looked at her and held back my tears, *oh shit, oh shit, oh shit*! I thought. *Here we go!*

17

The bus ride home was quiet. We were both in shock and it was neither the time nor place for an in depth discussion on the information we had just been given and I didn't know where to start so I kept quiet. Mum had gone someplace else, it was as though she had built a wall around herself which said, *enter at your own risk.*

I wasn't about to even knock on the door let alone enter, so I kept things to the mundane and asked, "what shall we have for dinner? What about fish with salad?"

"Ok!"

Well that was easy, I thought, *and safe.*

We had an early dinner, I did the dishes and sat down in Dad's chair facing the TV. Mum was staring out the window.

"Well Mum, I guess we wait for the appointment for your first chemo session?" I said venturing bravely into the territory which had been behind locked doors since seeing the Oncologist.

"I'm not making any decisions yet," she informed me. "I have a lot to think about and I have time to decide."

"Do you want to talk about your options?" I asked, moving further into 'trespassers will be shot' territory.

"There's not much to talk about! I either have chemo or not."

"You know you could come back to NZ with me," I offered, shaking inside at the thought of it, but also shaking at the thought of other options, more. Mum was not a problem to have around. It's just that she talked. Incessantly! Non stop! Hardly breathed between words!

And if she did happen to run out of words, she whistled, hummed, sang, anything to keep that noise coming out of her throat. It was amazing, exhausting, impressive and stressful. I remember coming home from a very hectic day at work when she was staying with me once and I stepped through the front door and it started. There was no down time, no cuppa with just silence to regroup. No, there was only a welcoming barrage of words.

I went to the toilet and sat there thinking it would give me 5, but no, the words were somehow defying physics and dematerialising only to materialise on the other side of the door, to penetrate my brain and keep the synapses firing, when all they wanted to do was shut down and sleep.

It took me back to when my children were little. I remember going to the toilet, not sure whether it was to be in my cave or for normal use, but I was on the loo and these little voices were coming through the door saying, "Mum, what are you doing?"

"I'm going to the toilet."

"Are you doing poos?"

"No, I'm just going wees."

"Are you going to be long?"

"No I'll be finished soon."

"Have you finished yet?"

Oh God, I thought, sitting there with my head in my hands thinking I can't even have a pee in peace! In fact it was more peaceful in their presence where they could see me, than in my little cubicle with the door shut between us.

I opened the door and burst into peals of laughter. There they were. My three sons and... the cat! Sitting on the floor, outside the toilet, as though a family meeting had been called.

It was hilarious and one of those moments that stays with you and brings a smile to your face when something triggers the memory.

That's how it was with Mum. She kept on keeping on as though she had a limited amount of time to be heard and she was cranking it along to get everything in.

"No", she said, decisively. "I am better off here with my things around me and stay in the hospital system that knows my history and has all my records."

"Ok, if you're sure? The offer stands at any time if you change your mind."

"Thanks, but I don't think I will."

18

We spent our days shopping for our meals, doing crosswords and watching TV. Mum who was an avid crossword fan had lost interest in doing them herself, but I noticed when I started to do them and got stuck, Mum was very good at helping me out. To keep her interest up and take her mind off things, especially something other than talking, I eventually involved Mum in every clue, which went something like this.

"10 across, 5 letters, clue is, cherub. Something n something, something l."

"Angel," she'd answer without any obvious signs of pondering on the clues.

"Yup, that fits," I'd say and move on to the next clue.

"12 across, 6 letters, clue is, a line of trucks. Something, something, n, something, o, y."

"Convoy," she'd come back with before my brain had engaged enough to even consider the positioning of the letters available.

Hell! I thought to myself after a while, I'm just taking dictation. My brain wasn't getting the workout it was drooling for. It was like showing a bone to a dog and then eating it yourself.

So to give myself a chance of actually answering some of the clues, I would make out I was looking for the next vacant spot in the crossword, but really I was checking out the next clue to see if I could answer it before giving it to Mum and opening the hatch for the falcon to swoop down and rip the answer from my pursed lips.

What a win/win I thought to myself, one crossword and two people getting enjoyment and kudos from the answers.

Every now and then both of us couldn't think of a word but we would always get there in the end and ploughed through at least a dozen or more of the magazines that a friend of Mum's had given her to help pass the days.

A couple of times we played the pokies, which was a pastime Mum had taken up to have a break from Dad when he was terminally ill. Mum would normally come away with some winnings even if it was only a few dollars. But lately her time on the pokies would eventuate in nothing but loss of her precious money and she would come away saying, "they're rigged. That's it, I'm not going back!" But she always would once she got bored enough.

As I wasn't sure how long I was going to be staying with Mum and before she started the chemo treatment, I decided I would get my hair cut and highlighted. It had been in Edinburgh a couple of months earlier that I had last been to a hairdresser, so I made an appointment for the following Monday, a few days before she was due to start her treatment. That way once she started the treatment I could be there for her and not have to think about when I could fit it in.

19

The weekend came and went with us only having a few quick trips to the shops to stock up on food. Mum bought her usual specials that would see her through to World War 3 and I followed in her wake, not wanting to upset her well established routine.

Monday morning came and Mum opened one of her several stocked cans of asparagus and spread it thinly across her toast. She sat in her chair facing the street and I sat in Dad's chair with my legs hanging over the arm closest to Mum. That way I could face her and listen to what she was saying.

"There goes hop-a-long," she said. "He probably fell off his motorbike and mangled his leg in the process. Damn motorbikes! Dangerous things! I don't know why they let them on the roads."

"Oh look at that, right on 5:30am. Mr Bentover, you could set your clock by him. He lost his wife not long ago you know, but he still gets out every morning without fail. I was a bit worried about him last week as he missed a few days, but he appeared again so must have got over his cold ok."

And so it went on. Once the morning traffic had settled into its rhythm, the kids came along going to kindy or school. She knew all of them as well. Not by name, but by one she had given them adopted from their appearance or actions. One little boy was her favourite. He would race along the street going hell-for-leather. He would be on a scooter, bike or just running with his head tilted back as though he was trying to catch the wind through his upturned nostrils. His pace was full tilt or stopped, there was nothing in between.

"Wheeeee," she'd say with a big smile on her face. "Look at him go. There'll be no stopping him in life!"

"S-o-o-n, that's it," I said, "all finished!" The clue was "Shortly", and that ended the second Colossus crossword in a row. "I'll make lunch and then I'm off to get my hair done."

"What would you like on your toasted sandwich?" It wasn't a matter of what to have for lunch. That was a given. It was just what filling to put in them that was the variant.

"Let's have the cheese with the onions and tomatoes," she replied enthusiastically. "I think that's my favourite. It's very tasty."

So off I went to the kitchen and made us each a toasted sandwich with the proverbial cup of tea and sat down on the sofa to eat lunch. Mum had swapped back to Dad's chair as the morning procession was over, so now she faced back into the room.

"Well, that's it I'm finished," I said, picking up my plate and cup and heading off to put them in the kitchen sink. "Time to watch *Last of the Summer Wine* and then I'll head off to the hairdresser."

"Do you want anything else before I head off to get my hair done?"

"No thanks, I'm ok for now."

"All right. I'll probably be at least a couple of hours. My hair is slow to take the colour so don't worry if I'm not back before 4pm." My appointment was for 1:30pm.

"Ok," she said. "Bye love."

"Bye Mum," and I closed the door behind me and set off to spend an few hours enjoying the peace and quiet of the salon.

I don't know about you, but whenever I get my hair done I can't wait to get home and wash out the style they've blow waved it in. What is it with hairdressers? Why do they make my hair look like I've just stepped out of a 60's movie? I just don't get it.

So as per usual after having my hair done, I headed off back to Mum's apartment at a brisk pace to get straight into the shower, and time warp myself back into present day reality.

I let myself in, with the usual, *I'm back,* only to be met with silence. I moved over to where I could see the back of Mum's chair, the one facing the street as it was obvious Dad's one facing into the room was empty. I knew immediately something was wrong. Her head was leaning forward, so from the back I could only see a small portion of the back of her head. A position she was never in.

Even when she fell asleep in the chair, her head was always leaning back, using the top the chair as a headrest.

I moved over to ease my way between the two chairs and I heard this cry come from deep within me and I burst into uncontrollable tears. "Mum! Oh God Mum! No! You should have told me. You should have let me know! You should have waited! You shouldn't have been on your own. It's not fair. Mum!" I held her face between my hands, she was cold. Her lips were blue and her mouth was partially open where the jaw had relaxed and released all the tension to allow it to drop.

Tears were streaming down my face and sobs racked my body as I held her and stroked her hair. It was so soft, so fine. I couldn't ever remember stroking Mum's hair. She looked so peaceful. Her legs were still crossed on the footstool. I knelt there sobbing, looking at my mother with incomprehensible sadness.

20

My sobs woke me up. *Oh shit! Oh shit! Oh shit! Please let it be a dream. Please! Please! Please,* I begged as I rolled out of bed and stumbled through blurred vision into the living room.

"You're up early," said a voice from behind the chair facing the street.

Oh God! I thought, wiping away the tears and preparing myself to act the part of someone who had just woken up from a peaceful night's sleep. T*hank you!*

"I've made a decision!" The chair said.

"Oooohhh!" I yawned to the back of the chair, trying to fake my relaxation as well as release the tension that had engulfed my body. I expected her to say, we'll go to Coles today, not Woolworths, as their asparagus is on special and I am running out. Mum had either asparagus or avocados on her toast for breakfast most mornings.

"Yes," the chair said, "I'm not having chemo."

So much for my habit of slowly, gently, easefully coming back into my body after a good night's sleep. It had been blown to smithereens twice. The tension which had been slowly sliding out of every cell, did a wheel spin and reversed back in, grasping hold of every cell and tightening until I was hyper alert, standing to attention and waiting for the bombshell that was about to hit.

"I'm taking my stuff," she informed me, as though she was passing on the morning weather report.

What do you say when your mother has just informed you she is going to end her life, after you've just faced her ending her life in a dream? My mind raced with all the options.

All the shouldn'ts, couldn'ts, mustn'ts and what abouts sat poised on my lips. But, this wasn't about me and my insecurities. It was about honouring my mother's right to choose. About honouring her decision and trusting that this 82 year old woman whose faculties were all in excellent working order, knew how and when she wanted to die. And what was more important, she was sharing it with me.

"Diane, I have lived a full life. I have experienced more than most people will ever experience in their lifetime. I have done everything I've ever wanted to do and there's nothing left I want to live for. Why put myself through the chemo, through anything that will maybe at best give me a few extra years. What for? There's nothing I want to do with them! Why experience the pain and suffering of chemo when it isn't going to cure anything and I will still have to die of something after all the struggle of trying to stay alive.

"Something's got to get me. Cancer, a stroke, heart attack or be run over by a bus. I can't see any point. It doesn't make any sense to try and live a little longer only to die a short while later. What sort of quality of life will I have in the interim? Nausea/vomiting, hair loss, dignity loss, diarrhoea/constipation, sore mouth, fatigue etc. etc. For God's sake I'm 82, I want to die peacefully! I've fought the fight the first time around and I did it to be with your father, then I fought his fight along with him and now he's gone I want to go to him.

"I've made up my mind! And I am not going to live what's left of my life watching the cancer slowly take over my body. The sooner I take my stuff the better. At least that way I will not be in a state of deterioration so as to be too weak to get myself out of here. This way I won't need to explain to anyone why I am not going to go ahead with any treatment."

Mum's face was set, jaw locked, eyes alert but distant. I had seen that look many times over the years. It meant don't question me, don't even suggest I'm wrong, you're wasting your time. My mind's made up.

I was quiet. Deathly quiet. There wasn't even an, "Oh shit" left in me. I surrendered.

"Are you sure?" I whispered, quietly, stoically. Knowing that from this moment forward, I had a choice to make that I would have to live with for the rest of my life.

"Yes", she affirmed with no hesitation what-soever.

"Then I'm going to stay with you," I answered back in the same quietly determined manner.

"You can't do that," she said whipping her head around and looking up at me with a question in her eyes.

"Oh yes I can," I replied. "No one deserves to die alone, no-one. This is my decision Mum. I have honoured yours, now you must honour mine.

"I will accept the consequences whatever they may be. They would never be as harsh as the ones I would have to live with if I left you to do this on your own."

I walked over to this strong but frail woman who had been in my life forever and put my arms around her and hugged her. We both cried.

It was the only time we allowed ourselves the freedom to feel the mass of emotions that encompassed the journey we were embarking on. A journey of mother and daughter saying goodbye. A journey where they both realised they were now equal in strength, equal in honour and respect, and equal in love.

21

After getting over the initial shock and having cleared my head as best as possible in the circumstances, I realised there was something I had to make clear to Mum before we went any further.

"Ok Mum," I said taking a deep breath in, "I'm your companion in this and I'll follow your lead. I will walk beside you and stay with you until the end, but there are some things I cannot have anything to do with. This is important to me so when it is over I know this is completely what you wanted and are responsible for, and that is the mixing, preparing and taking of your stuff."

"I understand," she replied nodding in agreement, "and just so you know, even if you weren't here I would do it anyway!"

"I know that Mum," I said out loud, *and I know why you're telling me,* I thought to myself.

"Ok Mum, talk me through it," I asked. "So I know what to expect and understand the process." Mum had been looking into euthanasia ever since Dad died so was well informed and had written everything down that she needed to remember. The only thing I wanted to know was how quickly it worked. I got on Google and found my answer. Thirty seconds to one minute to go unconscious and another minute for the heart to stop.

"Ok Mum," I said, "let's see if that time is acceptable," and set the stop watch on my iPhone. We sat looking at each other as the first 30 seconds ticked by and then one minute. It was a lifetime. "That's great," she said when the alarm went off. "Better than months of pain and agony and a slow lingering death."

She was truly prepared. Her notes said to have a small meal an hour before. Then half an hour before taking the Nembutal have a relaxant or sleeping pill. This was to help the body to relax and not reject the stuff by vomiting it up. Mix the stuff with orange juice or anything to make it palatable and have some mints or something strong tasting on hand to take away the bitter aftertaste.

"What have you got on hand to take afterwards?" I asked her?

"Not much," she said, "just these peppermints."

"I think we can do better than that Mum," I replied, thinking to myself this is going to be the last thing that passes her lips and it is not going to be some mouldy old peppermints.

"Let go across the road to the chocolate shop and get something delicious," I suggested and wasn't going to take no for an answer.

Amazingly she agreed, so off we went to the chocolate shop and after dragging her in, I left her to pick out the ones she liked. "Those ones there, they look good," she indicated, pointing to some dark chocolate-covered mint-centred ping-pong balls with flat bottoms. The girl with pink hair and matching nails informed us from colour co-ordinated pink lips, "they are $2.50 each."

"What?" Mum bellowed, nearly dropping dead on the spot. Which in retrospect may have saved us a lot of worry!

"I'm not paying that," she said, with a look of disgust and disbelief.

"You don't have to Mum, I'm buying them," I informed her, while she was still busy wallowing in indignation and I was busy trying to shrink myself into a ping-pong-sized person and blend in with the chocolates to avoid embarrassment.

"Mum! Why don't you wait outside while I get them," I said. Taking her by the arm and gently leading her away from the disgusting, decadent array of delicious, delightful, mouth watering treats.

I raised my eyebrows in disbelief. These were the last things my mother was ever going to taste and yet her World War 2 ration card was still firmly anchored in her psyche.

Oh God! I thought. *What a bloody shame that my mother is still stopping herself from having anything she considers extravagant, right up until the bitter end. (Pardon the pun)*

I splurged and bought three!

"Here Mum, try this," I insisted, pushing one into her mouth before she could say what a waste! "Better make sure you like them otherwise what's the point of replacing one disgusting taste with another?"

"Do you think they are strong enough to do the job?" I enquired raising my eyebrows.

"Yes," she muttered, through teeth now covered in that expensive, decadent, waste of money chocolate.

"Good," I said. "We've got two left. Do you think that's enough?" Of course that was a rhetorical question. I already knew the answer. I think one was more than enough in Mum's world.

"Plenty," she replied, as she quickly turned and headed off in the direction of home, just in case I came up with another expensive idea.

"Well that's everything, we've just got to set the date," she informed me as we walked into the apartment.

"And the sooner the better," she declared. "I don't want to even start chemo, so if I'm dead I won't need to give them an excuse why I'm not coming." She smiled, sounding very smug with herself over that fact.

Her first chemo appointment was for the following Thursday and it was Friday now.

"What about Monday?" I suggested. I always hated Mondays, so at least another day of the week wouldn't be tainted. Mondays would just keep on being what they already were. Crap!

"That's a good idea!" Mum agreed. "We can have a lovely weekend and then do it on Monday."

"What about one o'clock in the afternoon? We can have the morning to get ready, have lunch at twelve, sleeping pills at half past twelve and the stuff at one?"

"Ok! One o'clock Monday it is!" I affirmed.

"Mum is there anything you want to do over the weekend? Any place you want to visit?"

"No, I've done everything I wanted to do," she affirmed and I could vouch for that as my previous visit with Mum was like a trip down memory lane.

And so apart from the special lunch Mum had at one of her favourite restaurants, we continued on over the weekend with the same daily routine we had put in place over the weeks spent together. Breakfast, look out at the world passing on the street; morning tea, crosswords; lunch, TV;

afternoon tea reading; dinner, TV; evening cup of tea, bed.

In a blink of an eye it was Monday!

22

I don't know how to describe the feeling I had that morning when I awoke or actually when I decided it was time to get up. The night was long and sleep didn't even come close. It cowered in the corner holding tightly to its blanket of slumber.

I guess surreal is as good a word as any to describe the knowing in my gut that something momentous was about to happen and a sadness that it was.

Mum was quiet also. We had breakfast and looked out at the world going about its business in the street below. All her regulars went by. This was the last time she would comment on their walk, their appearance, their job, their parking and the reason they were out and about. They had no idea that this woman who had watched their evolution over the decades and who had given them a parallel life, was about to cease her commentary.

We did a few crosswords to pass the time and at twelve o'clock we had lunch. After lunch Mum went and got ready. She was calm, matter of fact and when she looked at me and saw I was close to tears, all she said was, "don't!" So I didn't! I sucked in and squeezed back all the emotion, all the grief and all the sadness that were on the edge threatening to spill over. They were mine to feel later I reasoned. *Don't,* the voice in my head echoed, *it's not about you,* it continued, *it won't help her.*

At half past twelve Mum pulled herself up out of her chair and informed me she was off to take her sleeping pill. They were ones that didn't knock her out, but just relaxed her enough for her to feel drowsy.

She took the two half packets of Nembutal powder and put them on the kitchen bench, along with a glass and a spoon.

The decadent, waste of money, extravagant, delicious, chocolates were put carefully beside her facing the street chair on her 'everything but the kitchen sink' table.

She sat down in her chair and quietly as if almost to herself she said, "I'm glad I can do this sitting here. I didn't want to be lying on my bed shut away in the bedroom. This way I can watch the world go by until the last minute. This has been my most favourite thing to do, second only to my walk."

"Mum, I need to ask this before you go any further, are you absolutely sure this is what you want? Are you positive you won't come back to NZ with me and be with the family?"

"What for Diane? It changes nothing! I still have cancer, I still either need treatment that will make my life miserable and will not cure me or let the cancer take over my body. I will still have to die of something! What happens if I get another clot and it paralyses me or I end up brain damaged? No, this is the way I choose to go. I'm doing it my way."

"Ok, Mum I just needed to be sure you weren't having any doubts or second thoughts?"

"Definitely not!" she replied getting up from her chair and saying as she walked into the kitchen, "I'll get the stuff ready."

I followed her into the kitchen and watched as she put the powder into the glass and filled it two thirds full with orange juice. The room echoed with the clinking noise as the spoon hit the sides of the glass on its frantic way around and around. All of a sudden I had a thought and blurted out, "don't lick the spoon." She stopped, turned and looked at me and we both burst out laughing.

"Right, that should do it," she said running water over the spoon to wash away any residue.

"It's time!"

Oh shit, oh shit, oh shit, I thought to myself, *this is it.*

We went back into the lounge and Mum put the glass on the side table while she got herself comfortable.

I knelt on the floor beside her chair so I could be near and hold her hand.

She put her legs up on her foot stool, wriggled back into her chair until she felt settled.

She picked up the glass, held it in the air and said, "right! Here we go!"

My stomach lurched, as I watched my mother down in a few gulps the liquid that was going to knock her unconscious and stop her heart.

"Urkkkk!" she mumbled and quickly put the glass down and picked up the chocolates, stuffing one immediately into her mouth, followed very quickly by the second one.

Then she sat back and waited. "It's not working", she said sounding extremely annoyed.

"Oh hold on, I can feel a coldness coming up my spine!"

I was holding her hand, tears were slowly escaping and trickling down my face. It was ok now to let go, she couldn't see them. "I love you Mum, thank you for being my Mum."

"I love you too," she whispered. "Thaaaank yoouuu fooorrrr staaayyyinng wiiitthhhh meeeeeeeee." Each word stretched out like a slow motion movie getting fainter and fainter until it vanished and her eyes closed and her head drooped forward.

23

I moaned and rolled over in bed. My pillow was cold on my cheek and I realised it was wet from my tears.

I sat up and swung my legs over the side of the bed, my toes curled into the carpeted floor as though they were gripping hold of something, anything, to stabilise my thoughts. Ever so hesitantly I stood and inched slowly expectantly towards the door. It was still dark which wasn't unusual as Mum's early morning routine was to sit in the twilight glow of the street lights and watch the world wake up.

I eased myself into the hallway and turned in the direction of the lounge. There was the chair, facing out to the street looking at a world not yet conscious, not yet transformed by that mellow aura of morning light from a sun sliding its way easefully towards the horizon. I stood transfixed to the back of that chair, waiting for her voice, waiting for a movement, waiting...

24

I remember coming home and plopping myself on the sofa and switching on the TV.

Ellen was interviewing Hugh Jackman. He was explaining his philosophy on dying alone (no, not euthanasia, just dying alone) and was saying, *I would rather die at 50 with my family and friends around me than have another 30 years of quality life and die alone at 80.*

I turned off the TV. I sat there with a myriad of thoughts swirling around in my head. Here is a virile man, has his health, isn't frail, isn't sick, and the last thing he would want for himself is to die alone. The thought is abhorrent to him.

I read an article in a newspaper once, where someone was arguing against euthanasia because it has been abused in the countries that had already legalised it. But isn't that the way of the world? Tell me one aspect of life that has not been abused. If you look back over the eons, every invention, law change, social policy, discovery, has been abused. There will always be a sector of humanity who will look for a way to take advantage of a situation, but do we stop the world turning because of this?

How do we tackle this problem? Certainly not by saying, "don't invent the wheel, it might cause accidents down the road!" No, we progress by trial and error. By seeing what works and what doesn't. We learn by our mistakes and to never have made any in the first place, is to never have extended ourselves or society as a whole.

Let's progress with our head and heart walking hand in hand into an enlightened place where suffering and pain are not seen as a flagellant's direct pathway to heaven. Where a decision can be made, legally with compassion, that a person has a right to say, *my time has come* and find a way that is painless, supportive and loving to celebrate their life and then say goodbye to it, surrounded by family, friends, compassion, joy and love.

Let them leave with these things in their hearts. Not emptiness, not guilt or shame and certainly not abandonment. How sad! How very sad, to make someone who is already suffering, suffer some more and die isolated and alone!

And how precious are those last words, *"thank you for staying with me!"*

THE END